Judith Morgan

Consultant Nurse

D1354236

Table of Contents

Preface

With few exceptions, the medical education system leaves budding clinicians to figure out clinical decision making on their own. In my years in the medical education process, both as a trainee and later as a teacher, I have seen few faculty give advice similar to what you will find in this book. Few written resources focus on the basics of clinical decision making. With time, most clinicians get to the point of making reasonable clinical decisions, but they may not understand how they arrive at their conclusions. The problem is this:

If they cannot evaluate their own processes, how can they hope to improve those same processes or hope to teach them effectively?

I think of this book as a letter to a younger me. This is the guide I wish I had during the early stages of my clinical training. I was not one of the trainees who intuitively understood how to make clinical decisions. I did not grasp the gist of it until I was already a senior resident. Initially I blamed my teachers for not teaching me the basics of clinical decision making However with time, and after talking with other colleagues, I realized that my teachers themselves were ignorant. Although good at teaching facts, they were ignorant of either the deeper processes of their own decision making or the need to teach decision making skills. In short:

Clinical decision making is a skill that every clinician uses but very few know how to teach.

After reading this book, hopefully clinical teachers will consider how to explain their own methods to their trainees. Often clinical teachers have intuited decision making throughout their career and have difficulty translating this skill into teachable form. Discussing something cognitive, abstract, and unseen allows us to analyze and improve upon it.

This book combines the rudimentary framework of decision making my teachers had inadvertently given me, lessons from reflecting upon my own clinical practice, my own experience as a clinical teacher, and my research into decision making. Putting all of this together, I developed a process that has worked well for me and my trainees. This book will show you this process.

Introduction

Clinical decision making is a skill that every clinician uses, but very few know how to teach. Many teachers are not explicitly aware of the need to teach this skill. Teaching facts and expanding on knowledge is much easier than coaching someone on the process of clinical decision making. Facts and knowledge are essential. However, they are only one part of the mental work that we do as clinicians. Without the analysis and critical thinking, those facts are **just data, not information**.

However, this mental work of clinical decision making the is at the core of medical practice. For many clinicians, the decision making process comes through experience alone, and not explicit instruction. To state this differently, clinical education is in essence an apprenticeship. It stems from the tried and true medical tradition of "see one, do one, teach one" or as I prefer to describe it, "monkey see, monkey do." In a skilled craftsman's apprenticeship, the apprentice tries to mimic the teacher's methods until they mimic the skills to the teacher's satisfaction. This works well when the trainee can literally see the skill to mimic, for example: carpentry.

But what happens if the skill is cognitive? It is difficult to see a skill that is inside someone's mind. We can see how to use a hammer on a nail, but we have a more difficult time seeing how to use decision making processes to diagnose appendicitis. The skill is mental, and mental work cannot be seen and mimicked.

Consider the hypothetical case of a 30-year-old female who complains of pleuritic chest pain, for instance:

- A third year medical student sees the patient, spends about 20 minutes taking a comprehensive history and physical. He collects as much data as possible to try to make sense of what is going on. By the end, he has a vague idea of the patient's differential diagnosis, and is even less sure of a plan.

- <u>A first year resident</u> sees the patient, spends about 10 minutes taking a history and physical exam. She focuses more than the medical student and tries to collect as much supporting data as possible. She believes the patient has a pulmonary embolism. She considers imaging and bloodwork.
- <u>The attending physician</u> sees the patient, spends about 5 minutes taking a focused history and physical exam. She quickly deduces that the patient has costochondritis and rules out other, more serious causes of pain. She recommends NSAIDs and discharge home.

In rounds, the attending explains the key aspects of why the patient had costochondritis and not a pulmonary embolism to the medical student and resident. Although a seasoned clinician and expert explainer of medical facts, the attending does not actually discuss *the process* of making the diagnosis itself. Often, she cannot explain how she achieved this diagnosis. Instead, she offers her trainees the tried-and-true advice that their diagnostic skills will improve with experience and more studying.

The attending herself believes this; this is how her mentors trained her, and this is how she trains her own trainees. To this attending, clinical decision making is something that naturally evolves with diligence, time, and experience. However, it may also remain a mysterious black box that somehow gives us a reasonable differential diagnosis in the end.

On one level, the attending is right: the trainees' diagnostic skills will indeed improve with time. Virtually all clinical trainees eventually become competent clinical decision makers, but trainees essentially stumble their way through learning the decision making processes.

On another level, this traditional method can be a painful experience. Trainees receive little concrete feedback on the process itself. The underlying processes for making clinical decisions may not be understood. If trainees did understand these processes, they would most likely mature more quickly as clinicians.

But there is an even more important reason to understand decision making processes: The patient's health is at stake. **Understanding the processes may decrease the probability of trainees making decision-making mistakes.**

In this book, I am going to discuss a framework for making clinical decisions. With this framework, trainees can have both a reference point and a method for feedback on their decision making skills.

Specifically, this approach addresses clinical decision making from a perspective that is more closely related to **the art of medicine** than that of the science. As with other arts, a teacher gives skills and guidance, but students have the responsibility to put the art into practice and make it their own. I will approach the art of clinical decision making systematically as a teachable skill.

<u>What this book is:</u>

This book is primarily a guide for <u>medical trainees</u>. For the purpose of this book, 'medical trainees' include medical students, residents, physician assistant students, and nurse practitioner students.

Additionally, clinical teachers should find this book useful as a teaching tool.

Ideally, this book is:

> <u>A tool.</u> This will provide trainees with a basic start for clinical decision making. Once you have some experience using these tools, you should be ready to delve into the more technical aspects of clinical decision making and be better able to explore the methods of other teachers.

> <u>A user-friendly manual</u>. You will be able to use some of these tools *right out of the box*. However, you still have to explore the tools and principles on your own.

> <u>A guide</u>. This book should be like a good teacher. A good teacher opens the way for the students, but does not take them to their destination.[Confucius p247] Think of this work as a guide to help keep you on track. But note, **you have to make the journey yourself**.

I hope that after reading this book, both teachers and trainees will reflect on their own processes, dissect them, discuss them, and become better decision makers.

What this book is not:

Simply put, this book is <u>not</u>:

> <u>An end.</u> It does not represent the totality of what clinical decision making is about. It is a basic beginning, a primer. Furthermore, I will not pretend that the method illustrated is the only or best way to go about making these decisions. The method I demonstrate is the basic method of **my way**, which I developed through experience, research, and trial and error. This method and process works for me and works for my trainees. Others teachers may have different processes, **and that is fine**.

> <u>A magic bullet.</u> This book will not make you a master clinical decision maker merely by reading it. As with any art, you must practice what you learn.

> <u>Medical decision making through applied statistics.</u> Those methods are beyond the scope of our discussion. There are many fine resources for a more mathematical analysis of decision making. I have used some of them in researching this book and have included a few in the bibliography.

> <u>A **science of medicine** perspective</u>. Again, what I will explore is closer to the **art of medicine**.

Even with these caveats, one can approach decision making systematically and as a teachable skill.

What is clinical decision making?

At the most basic level, clinical decision making is one aspect of the art of medicine. It is **mental work** that is **applied to a clinical situation**. This is the core of what clinicians do. This mental work **involves critical thinking**, which is:

- Reflecting on assumptions and beliefs,
- Critiquing self-thought and action,
- Hunting assumptions,
- Checking assumptions, and
- Seeing things from different viewpoints.[Merriam p214]

Clinical decision making combines critical thinking with medical knowledge in order to form a list of possible diagnoses (a differential diagnosis) for the purpose of creating and carrying out a treatment plan. Statistics and evidence are part of a toolbox that clinical decision makers use in their craft.

Clinical decision making therefore uses <u>knowledge as a tool</u>.

It follows that we clinicians are *knowledge workers*, wherein knowledge and training are our tools.[Drucker p37] Our value lies in our ability to use these tools in order to achieve our desired outcome, namely: healthier patients. We have the tools and the methods to use them in our minds. In a sense, we own the means of production.[Drucker p38]

Our Cognitive Tools

Our cognitive tools for clinical decision making include heuristics and Bayes' theorem. Later, I will apply them in depth to several examples.

Heuristics: Definition, advantages, and cautions
Heuristics are **cognitive processes** that:

- Are used to learn, recall, or understand knowledge,[Sox p37]
- **Function as rules of thumb,**[Sox p37]
- Simplify decision making processes,[Weingart p61]
- Describe everyday intuitive decisions without formal decision making processes.[Weingart p61]

A simple non-clinical example of a heuristic is that lots of dark clouds overhead suggests that it is going to rain.

A simple medical example is that right lower quadrant tenderness with rebound suggests appendicitis.

Clinicians rely heavily on heuristics, and for the most part they are accurate.[Kassirer p5]

That being said, heuristics are powerful tools that we must use with care. Improperly used, heuristics can reflect a person's bias and lead to mistakes in decision making.[Sox p37, Weingart p61] We can decrease our chance of error by being systematic in our usage.[Hunkink p402]

Heuristics work best when adapted to a specific task,[Newell p75] but often, we have to apply our heuristics to new situations. In such cases, we have to 'substitute attributes,' or replace an attribute in the current problem with a likely-related attribute in a known heuristic.[Newell p75-76] We place **a new value into an old framework,** hoping that the new value will be a close-enough approximation for the old one. For example, if you have a patient in front of you with chest pain, you will most likely draw from experiences with other similar patients in order to help you arrive at diagnoses and treatment plans.

In a clinical setting, you can think of every new patient encounter as an attribute substitution, but with some caution. We may recall a patient that is similar to the one we are currently treating and hope that the two cases are close enough that the heuristic that we had used for the old patient will work for the new one. However, the two patients' situations may be different enough that attribute substitution does not work. This mismatch is one of the risks of attribute substitution: we may give the right answer to the wrong question.[Newell p80]

Of the many heuristics that clinicians use, I will discuss three heuristics in our cognitive toolbox:

- **Availability**
- **Representativeness**
- **Anchoring and adjustment.**

Availability Heuristic: Definition and limits

With the **availability heuristic**, people judge the probability of an event with how easily they remember it.[Sox p47] People tend to recall an event if some aspect of the disease makes it easy to remember. For example, people recall unusual events more easily than mundane ones.[Hunkink p141]

Other factors that affect availability are frequency, recentness, and vividness.[Sox pp48-49] For example, if you saw a patient with a pheochromocytoma yesterday, you might suspect it in the next patient that you see with an elevated blood pressure, even though pheochromocytomas are rare.

A major limit to the availability heuristic is the extent of your own knowledge. If you don't know about a condition or its treatment, you won't know to consider it. Several of my teachers told me that if you don't know about a disease, you're never going to see it. **So you need a good <u>knowledge base</u> in order to use the availability heuristic well.**

Representativeness Heuristic: Definition and limits

The **representativeness heuristic** is an event's probability determined by how closely the patient's picture matches a *typical picture* for a disease.[Hunkink p141-142] Other terms to describe the representativeness heuristic are **pattern recognition** or **illness scripts**.

An example of the representativeness heuristic is a mental model of what a patient with cholecystitis should look like: a patient with right upper quadrant tenderness, fever, vomiting, and a positive Murphy's sign.

Limits of the representativeness heuristic include:

1. Not taking into account the probability of a disease in a given population.
2. Clinical findings may not accurately predict the disease.
3. Symptoms may typically appear together regardless of the disease.
4. Sample size is too small, such as a sample derived solely from personal experience.[Sox P37-47]

Anchoring and Adjustment Heuristic: Definition and limits

The **anchoring and adjustment heuristic** is an initial probability judgement (the anchor) of a particular disease that is then shaped into a final estimate, after taking the individual patient's characteristics into account (the adjustment).[Sox p49]

For instance, if your initial impression was that a patient had streptococcal pharyngitis (your anchor), additional information (adjustment) could change your diagnosis.

Limits to the anchoring and adjustment heuristic include two potential traps:

1. Setting the initial anchor incorrectly, and
2. Not adjusting correctly for new information.[Sox p49]

Beware: information obtained after setting the anchor is very influential.[Hunkink p400] You may find it difficult to change your anchor once you have set it.

Using published evidence to set the anchor can minimize error when anchoring. Published evidence presents a wider body of evidence — a larger sample size — than your individual experience.[Sox p52] As you obtain new information, give it its appropriate weight.

Bayes' Theorem: Definition and limits
Bayes' theorem helps clarify the anchoring and adjustment heuristic.

Bayes' theorem, a complex mathematical model, is that **new information about a patient's condition changes our probability of the disease being present.**[Sox p5] As a model, the theorem indicates how much to change a probability based on new information, specifically the probability of a disease being present **before** a test (pre-test probability) and the probability of a disease **after** a test (post-test probability). Each new bit of information changes our estimated probability of disease by a certain amount. Intuitively, this makes sense and is very useful in clinical decision making.

While a full explanation of the theorem is beyond the scope of our discussion, the basic concept is valuable for clinical decision making and is related to the anchoring and adjustment heuristic:

The clinical picture can change as we add new information.

For example, we would change our initial diagnosis of cholecystitis once the ultrasound indicates a normal gallbladder but an enlarged liver.

Limits to Bayes' Theorem:

1. Unfortunately, the formula of Bayes' theorem is too complicated to use in many real-life clinical settings.[Hunkink p136] Instead, people tend to use short cut solutions, basically heuristics.[Newell p77]
2. A naïve approach to Bayes' theorem assumes that each piece of evidence is independent.[Newell p72] Symptom #1 might directly lead to symptom #2. The disease may not directly cause symptom #2. So if symptoms #1 and #2 are both present, the probability of the disease does not increase, e.g.:

> Nausea and vomiting. Vomiting almost always comes with nausea. Do not treat them as independent factors.

3. People tend to embrace reasons that support their views and ignore reasons that support opposing views, e.g.:[Newell p88]

    > If you are considering a myocardial infarction as a patient's diagnosis, you only look for evidence that supports myocardial infarction, and not evidence for an alternate diagnosis, such as pulmonary embolism or aortic dissection.

4. Different pieces of information have different weights. Beware of overweighting unlikely probabilities and underweighting likelier ones, e.g.:[Newell p127]

    > An infiltrate on a chest x-ray in a patient with suspected pneumonia likely has more weight than a clear lung auscultation.

In everyday life, professionals rely on a combination of representativeness and availability heuristics[Newell p198], and the underlying concepts of the Bayes' Theorem. The next step is to use them in a systematic process in order to obtain a diagnosis.

Obtaining a Diagnosis

To obtain a diagnosis, clinicians infer the possible causes of the symptoms.[Kassirer p5] We gather data, interpret data, begin probing possible solutions, decide on an appropriate solution, and confirm the decision. Clinical decision making is thus part detective work and part problem solving.

One of the hard parts about obtaining a correct diagnosis is the uncertainty inherent in medical practice. **Medicine is the <u>art</u> of making clinical decisions without adequate information.**[Sox p ix, emphasis added] Often we must act without knowing with 100% certainty whether a disease is present. In short, we must use our best estimate, and arriving at a best estimate is a process. The processes that we use are therefore important to know and understand.

In order to decrease the inherent uncertainty in the art of medical decision making, we apply the three heuristics and Bayes' Theorem to stages of the process of obtaining a diagnosis.

The Process of Obtaining a Diagnosis

We will use the three heuristics in the following order:

1. Availability
2. Represenativeness
3. Anchoring and Adjustment

In the real world, these processes often are intertwined. You will do them simultaneously and often repeatedly. With experience, these processes work faster than you might think, compared to when you first learned them. You may go through them several times, just to obtain the history. In this section, I will break down the process into smaller, separate ones for ease of discussion, and then apply them to examples.

Part I: Apply a version of the **availability heuristic**

Have a few diagnoses in mind when you go into a patient encounter. Expert clinicians often generate their hypotheses early in the encounter, but why they do so matters.[Sox p10] These clinicians are not merely data gathering. Rather, **they are testing the probabilities of their hypotheses.**[Sox p12]

I will mirror this process. How do we pick the diagnoses?

1. **Consider what is:**
   - Most likely
   - Most dangerous.

   The most dangerous possibilities are usually straightforward. What is most likely sometimes takes a little more consideration.

2. **For the *most likely* possibility, ask yourself:**
   - What are the likely diagnoses in this patient's part of the population?
   - Is this patient at particularly high risk for certain diagnoses?

   You can draw on personal experience, general medical knowledge, and specific published data in order to choose the diagnoses to test.

Part II: Test your possible diagnoses via history and physical exam using the **representativeness heuristic**

Match the patient's findings with a mental model or picture of what the disease should look like. This process is **pattern recognition**.

Two analogies can help you visualize this part of the process:

- **Think: pieces of a puzzle**. Try to see how well the patient before you matches the disease that you have in mind. When you have enough pieces together, take the proverbial step back and see how they fit. If they fit pretty well, you may have the diagnosis. If they do not, you may have to consider another diagnosis.
- **Think: a scale**. Add evidence for or against a diagnosis on either side of the mental scale in order to see which side has more evidence and is therefore the weightier argument.

*Part III: Keeping the concept of Bayes' Theorem in mind, use a version of the **anchoring and adjustment** heuristic.*

If you find that a particular diagnosis fits pretty well with your initial information gathering, then investigate its likelihood further. In other words:

1. Once you set your **anchor**,
2. Gather new information.
3. See how much it changes the picture of what is going on with your patient, and then
4. See what kind of **adjustments** you have to make with the additional information at hand.

Think of anchoring and adjustment as a Bayesian concept: adjust the probability of the disease as you gain new information about the patient. You may visualize this as a mental scale wherein the new information you gather will either work for or against the anchored diagnosis.

Minimizing Bias

Think of a bias as something that might sway your clinical decision in one direction or another without really having sufficient weight to do so.

I will briefly discuss three strategies to minimize bias and improve your ability to make correct decisions:

1. **Question your own conclusion.**[Newell p246] Ask yourself, "What evidence points away from my conclusion?"

2. **Continue searching for an answer after you have reached that preliminary conclusion.**[Newell p 248] Ask yourself, "Is there a better explanation?"

3. **Do not fear the *sunk cost* effect.** The *sunk cost* effect is the tendency to continue a plan in which one has invested resources, even after the plan has been revealed as irrational.[Newell p189] If the sensible course of action is to change the plan, then do so, despite initially investing time and energy in another direction. Thankfully, the temptation to give in to the *sunk cost effect* diminishes with expertise.[Newell p189-190]

Think of these strategies in relation to the anchoring and adjustment heuristic. Ask yourself whether you have anchored in the right place, and do not be afraid to pull up anchor if you find yourself in the wrong place.

Arriving at the Diagnosis: Applying the Process to Methods of Obtaining Information

The patient history gives us information for narrowing down the diagnosis, just like the physical exam and testing. All of these methods provide us clinicians with information, and thus, we can apply the same processes.

In this and the following examples, we will start out with two diagnoses, but you could use however many diagnoses you are comfortable remembering while you begin to evaluate the patient. **Although the process can seem slow at first, with practice it will speed up a lot.** The purpose is to help us gain **more** information in a **targeted fashion.**

PATIENT HISTORY:

Example #1: 30-year-old male with abdominal pain.

Step 1: Modified Availability Heuristic

Even with this small amount of information, we can generate diagnoses to test. Let's pick a couple diagnoses to tests: pancreatitis and appendicitis.

Step 2: The Representativeness Heuristic

Keep in mind the expected symptom pattern of each disease. We are actively looking for evidence for and against each disease. Ask about symptoms of both in order to see how much evidence we have for either one.

Our initial lists could look something like this:

Pancreatitis	**Appendicitis**
Vomiting	Vomiting
Nausea	Nausea
Light colored stool	Poor appetite
History of heavy alcohol drinking	Worse with movement
Left upper quadrant pain	Right lower quadrant pain
Pain radiates to the back	Pain starts near the umbilicus and then migrates to the right lower quadrant

We ask some initial questions based on the lists that we have in mind, testing to see how likely either diagnosis is.

The patient confirms vomiting, nausea, poor appetite, and right lower quadrant pain. The patient said no to every other symptom on the list. Appendicitis seems more likely than pancreatitis. However, we have to investigate further.

Our lists now look like this:

<u>Pancreatitis</u>	**<u>Appendicitis</u>**
Vomiting	Vomiting
Nausea	Nausea
███████████	Poor appetite
███████████	███████████
███████████	Right lower quadrant pain
███████████	███████████

Step 3: Anchoring and Adjustment Heuristic

We gather more information in order to adjust our probability of appendicitis by asking more questions about appendicitis. Often we have to elicit this evidence directly. Other times the patient will volunteer this evidence during the history. After a certain point, there will be so much evidence **for or against** that it will take a considerable weight of evidence to tip the mental scales in the other direction. As we continue to talk, the patient tells us that:

- o His pain extends to his right flank.
- o Urinating makes his pain worse.
- o He has had this pain on and off for months but never got checked for it.

Now we have evidence against appendicitis and for another diagnosis. The patient's clinical picture is now suspicious for a kidney stone.

We should repeat the same steps that we have outlined above in order to evaluate for a kidney stone, starting with the representativeness heuristic (in this case, a list of expected symptoms for a kidney stone). We should test how well the patient's symptoms fit the symptom pattern of a kidney stone.

Example # 2: A 40-year-old woman complains of chest pain. She is post-operative day #1 after a cholecystectomy. She has no other medical history.

Step 1: Availability Heuristic

We will consider pulmonary embolism and myocardial infarction as the first two possibilities to test.

Step 2: Representativeness Heuristic

Make a mental list of the expected findings and then test them against the patient's symptoms. Our initial list may look something like this:

Pulmonary Embolism	Myocardial Infarction
Pain may or may not radiate.	Pain radiates to the left arm.
Shortness of breath	Shortness of breath
History of recent surgery	History of hypertension and/or diabetes
Any location on the chest	Left sided
Sharp	Heavy
Pleuritic	Non-pleuritic

When we speak with the patient, we can match the symptoms against both lists to see which set pairs better. We will then have an anchoring diagnosis to further test.

Let's say the patient tells us her chest pain is right sided, pleuritic, sharp, and comes with shortness of breath. No pain radiation, history of hypertension, or history of diabetes. She has the beginnings of a pretty good story for a pulmonary embolism.

Our lists now look like this:

Pulmonary Embolism	Myocardial Infarction
███████	███████
Shortness of breath	Shortness of breath
History of recent surgery	███████
Any location on the chest	███████
Sharp	███████
Pleuritic	███████

Step 3: Anchoring and Adjustment

Using pulmonary embolism as our working diagnosis, we will obtain more information in order to confirm it. This can come through additional history. For example, we can ask her if she has leg swelling, leg pain, recent travel, or takes oral contraceptives.

Later, we may get additional information via the physical exam or testing, both of which we will also subject to our heuristics.

> Remember the analogy of a scale? This new information can add or subtract weight to the argument that this patient has a pulmonary embolism.

Alternatively, remember the analogy of a puzzle? The new information may give us more pieces to build a more complete picture.

As we have already discussed, if the evidence is overwhelming for or against, you will need compelling evidence to the contrary in order to significantly change the probability.

Caveat about Obtaining Patient History: How to Handle Interference Answers

Interference answers are when a patient answers a different question than the one you asked. This is a common occurrence. Here are some examples of interference answers:

You	Patient
What brings you in today?	My doctor's office is on 31st street.
When did your abdominal pain start?	My left foot has a rash.
How strong is your leg pain?	I get twitching in my neck sometimes.

Answers like these can throw a clinician off track, so:

1. Keep your possible diagnoses in mind; you will be less likely to be thrown off by interference answers.
2. Maintain your focus on assessing your initial potential diagnoses <u>before</u> tracking down the information the patient gives you.
3. Follow up on what the patient mentions in the inference answers because sometimes, <u>that</u> ends up being the patient's true concern.

Doing these things will keep your focus clear while still paying keen attention to your patient's concerns.

PHYSICAL EXAM:

The history will often narrow the possible diagnoses, and sometimes it will give you the diagnosis without need for further evidence. Other times, we must collect information in other ways, such as the physical exam.

For the physical exam, I will use **the same process** outlined for the history.

The physical exam starts the moment that you lay eyes on the patient. We should observe our patient closely and keep in mind the expected findings of the patient's potential diagnoses.

Example # 1: 65-year-old male with vague abdominal pain worsening for about 1 week. His previous history is of hypertension and alcohol abuse.

Step 1: Availability heuristic

We will consider gastritis and hepatitis for this example.

Step2: Representativeness Heuristic

A list of preliminary expected findings could include:

Gastritis	Hepatitis
Epigastric tenderness	Right upper quadrant tenderness
Normal skin	Jaundice
Normal eyes	Icterus
Normal sized liver	Enlarged liver
	Spider nevi

When you examine the patient, look specifically for the above findings from the start.

Your exam finds right upper quadrant tenderness, mild jaundice, and mild icterus. There is a normal sized liver, no other tenderness, and no spider nevi.

Our list now looks like this:

Gastritis	Hepatitis
▮▮▮▮▮▮▮▮▮▮	Right upper quadrant tenderness
▮▮▮▮▮	Jaundice
	Icterus
Normal sized liver	▮▮▮▮▮
	▮▮▮▮▮

Step 3: Anchoring and adjustment

Our preliminary (anchoring) diagnosis is now hepatitis. We should look for other findings during our physical exam in order to add to or subtract from the probability that the patient has hepatitis: asterixis or an irregularly shaped liver, for instance. Based on those findings, hepatitis will be more or less likely. When combined with other sources of information, such as history and testing, we will have a pretty good estimate of the likelihood of hepatitis.

If we find more evidence confirming hepatitis, then we may proceed with treatment. However, if we find significant evidence contrary to hepatitis, we can throw out that diagnosis and set a new anchor.

Example # 2: 12-year-old female with left leg pain and swelling. Symptoms started after she tripped and fell. She has no past medical history.

Step 1: Modified Availability Heuristic

We will consider the initial possible diagnoses of fracture and contusion.

Step 2: Representativeness Heuristic

A possible list of initial physical exam findings might include:

Fracture	Contusion
Point tenderness at fracture	Diffuse tenderness at injury
Large amount of swelling	Medium to small amount of swelling
Bony deformity to the leg	No deformity to the leg
Looks very uncomfortable	Looks mildly uncomfortable

With the above mental lists in mind, we go see the patient. We find a 12-year-old girl who looks very uncomfortable with diffuse tenderness to her site of injury and large amounts of swelling. You cannot tell if there is a bony deformity because there is so much swelling. Although the picture is mixed, more factors weigh towards fracture.

Our lists might now look something like this:

Fracture	Contusion
	Diffuse tenderness at injury
Large amount of swelling	
Looks very uncomfortable	

Step 3: Anchoring and Adjustment Heuristic

We have anchored on fracture as our working diagnoses. We should try to collect more information in order to increase or decrease the likelihood that her injury is a fracture, such as severe pain when she moves the extremity or whether she can walk.

A case like this shows that **additional information can be a tie breaker**. Imagine a mental scale instead of the above list, if you prefer. On one side of the scale is the fracture, and on the other side is the contusion. Additional information is very useful for tipping the mental scale towards one diagnosis or the other and can come from further history, physical exam details, or testing.

TESTING:

We can apply the same process to testing that we have used for other data gathering processes, such as the history and the physical exam, but first I will address a few points because so many people misunderstand testing's proper function.

Medical testing has a certain mystique for patients and some clinicians as well. **Sadly, many people think that without tests, there is no information. These people are wrong.** For clinicians especially, tests should **not** cause this kind of fascination.

Some proper functions of tests include:

1. Providing information that the history and physical exam cannot.
2. Helping to narrow down possible diagnoses.
3. Demonstrating effectiveness of treatment over time.
4. Determining the extent of disease.
5. Estimating a patient's prognosis.

Tests are just another source of data for you to use when making a clinical decision. We often use them after we have already obtained information from a history and physical exam. The data that tests provide are just one piece of the puzzle that is your patient. Tests help us complete the puzzle of what is going on with the patient and can become a tie breaker in some cases, but they rarely give the whole picture. In fact, they can have several limitations.

Some limitations of tests:

- **Tests require interpretation; clinicians must give the results meaning.** Make the test's data useful. A quote from a business management text sums up nicely the difference between data and information: "Information is data endowed with relevance and purpose."[Drucker p271] Your knowledge base and critical thinking skills transform data into information. The test result by itself does <u>not</u> give you the answer.

- **Tests can be wrong.** The tests we use in medicine are very good, but they are not perfect. All tests have false positives or false negatives.[Weingart p32] Even a test considered the *gold standard* for a disease can be wrong.[Weingart p33]

- **The same test result can mean different things in different contexts.** Think about the overall picture when interpreting test results. Ask yourself, "How does this piece of information fit into the puzzle that is our patient?" For example, a white blood cell count of 15,000:

  - Adds evidence that the patient's pneumonia is **getting worse** if the patient has a worsening cough, high fever, and a white blood cell count of 12,000 yesterday.

  - Adds evidence that the patient's pneumonia is **getting better**, when the patient had been admitted for pneumonia for several days, had a white blood cell count of 20,000 yesterday, and has no fever today.

- **Tests run risks.** Tests are not benign. Tests can delay treatment, cost a lot of money, or cause direct harm to your patient.[Hunkink p158]

Therefore, consider both the benefits and costs of tests when you order them. Ask yourself the following question *before* ordering:

1. <u>How much will this test result change the big picture?</u> In essence, this question asks you to anticipate the results of applying Bayes' theorem, and the anchoring and adjustment heuristic, since new information can change the probability of the disease, namely: how much will the test result affect your expected probability of a disease being present (the post-test probability).

2. <u>Will this test make a difference?</u> If the result will not push the clinician past the threshold to either initiate or withhold treatment, then you should not do the test.[Hunkink p148]

For instance:

o You suspect appendicitis in a patient with right lower quadrant pain for two days, loss of appetite, vomiting, mild fever, and right lower quadrant tenderness with guarding. You have quite a bit of evidence for appendicitis already. Is a white blood cell count going to significantly change your expected probability of appendicitis?

o You suspect either a hemorrhagic stroke or post seizure paralysis in a patient who had a dull headache followed by a seizure. He is now very sleepy, mumbling incoherently, not following commands, and does not move his right arm. The evidence you have so far can go either way. In this case, we need an information tiebreaker. Can a CT scan of the head give evidence that will swing the diagnosis one way or the other?

Interpreting new data depends on what we already know about the patient.[Sox p84] **We should not order or interpret test results in a vacuum**. Consider the context of the situation when you think about ordering a test.

Specifically, we can apply a **version of the process** we have already used with the history and the physical examination to tests, but we must add another dimension: **risk**.

Example #1: A 70-year-old man has a history of hypertension and an abdominal aneurysm that is three cm in diameter. He has no acute symptoms. His last evaluation for the aneurysm was six months ago. In order to monitor him for possible increase in aneurysm diameter, we must screen him.

Step 1: Availability Heuristic
In terms of testing, we can think of this as which tests we have available. For this case, we will consider CT scan and ultrasound.

Step 2: Representativeness Heuristic
We start by listing the expected characteristics of each test. From this list we will start to determine which test is better suited for this situation. **Some tests will be better for certain situations than others.** This analysis includes the advantages, disadvantages, and limitations of each test.

A list for this patient can look like this:

CT scan	Ultrasound
Visualizes the aorta well	Usually visualizes the aorta well
Visualizes other internal organs	Bowel gas can interfere
Easier to interpret	Operator dependent
Radiation	No radiation
Intravenous contrast can injure kidneys	Does not need intravenous contrast
Intravenous contrast can cause allergic reaction	

Step 3: Anchoring and Adjusting Heuristic with Risk

The way we apply the anchoring and adjusting heuristic here is a bit different from the previous steps in the process. A simple way to think about it is this: we have two anchors, one on each side of the scale. Both tests have different risks and different benefits. We must weigh the pros and cons of both choices. Risks subtract from the weight. Benefits add to the weight. When we've adjusted each side with risks and benefits, then we can decide which of the two tests has more value.

Alternatively, we can imagine crossing factors off of the lists of test characteristics, based upon the patient's situation.

In this case, the patient's history may add weight one way or the other. For example, a patient with kidney disease will be a poor candidate for a CT scan, while an obese patient may be a poor candidate for an ultrasound.

The patient's specific characteristics will further define which test will be the better choice. They can function as additional weight on your mental scale.

Example #2: A 37-year-old female with a history of alcohol abuse comes in for abdominal pain and vomiting. She is uncomfortable and has epigastric tenderness. She has no jaundice or icterus. You consider alcoholic gastritis versus pancreatitis.

Step 1: Availability heuristic

You consider differentiating by obtaining a serum lipase. You cannot think of another alternative.

Step 2: Representativeness Heuristic

A serum lipase is specific, reliable, and easy to obtain.

Step 3: Anchoring and Adjustment Heuristic

The test result indicates that lipase is elevated. This adds a lot of weight to the probability of pancreatitis.

After discussing with your colleagues, you decide to go one step further and obtain further testing. You decide that the patient's pancreas needs imaging. You intend for the imaging to add more evidence for pancreatitis, its extent, and possible complications (especially pseudocysts), and repeat the process in order to determine which type of imaging is the most productive.

Step 1: Availability Heuristic

You consider an abdominal ultrasound and abdominal X-ray in order to visualize the pancreas.

Step 2: Representativeness Heuristic

Possible lists of characteristics might look like this:

Ultrasound	X-ray
Typically visualizes pancreas well	Good for bony structures
Visualizes soft tissue well	Limited visualization of soft tissue
Bowel gas can limit quality	May visualize pancreatic calcifications
No radiation	Radiation
Good at visualizing pseudocysts	Poor at visualizing pseudocysts

You decide that the ultrasound is the better test overall.

Step 3: Anchoring and Adjustment Heuristic

The ultrasound shows the entire pancreas is swollen and inflamed. No signs of pseudocysts. You now have more evidence for pancreatitis and against its complications.

You wonder if you have enough information or need more in order to adjust the probability of pancreatitis. A colleague mentions that a CT scan with IV contrast is a better method of imaging the pancreas than ultrasound.

Even if the CT scan is better at finding pancreatitis, ask yourself:

- What additional details could a CT scan provide in order to improve the diagnosis?
- Will CT scan results change the care the patient will receive?
- What risks does a CT scan have?

- After balancing the risks of the CT scan with the possible benefits, which has more weight on your mental scale?

I will leave these questions for you to consider.

Finally, consider these three summarizing points by Sox regarding testing:

> **If a disease is very certain, do not test and do treat.**
> **If a disease is very unlikely, do not test and do not treat.**
> **If probability of disease is intermediate, consider testing.**[Sox p33]

Implications of a Diagnosis

Arriving at a diagnosis is just one part of your work as a clinician. What you do with that diagnosis directs your care of your patient via your treatment plan, but only in so far as you can communicate it effectively to others. I will consider both elements separately.

Making a Treatment Plan

By the time we clinicians are considering making a treatment plan, we have already acquired a lot of data about our patient and analyzed it critically. **By this point, we should have a single, working diagnosis.** In a sense, we have completed the hardest part. Typically, when we have a diagnosis, knowing what to do is easier. <u>Your treatment plan will spring from your diagnosis.</u>

Often, simply reading from a textbook passage regarding your diagnosis will tell you what to do, but **there are still some very important concepts you should be aware of** in making your plan.

Have Clear Objectives

We clinicians have to make what we are trying to achieve explicit.[Hunkink p5] Have clear objectives before carrying out your plan.[Hunkink p7] Without a clear goal, you will likely waste time and effort.

Ask yourself:

1. What is the goal of our treatment? Examples include:
   - Controlling pain
   - Improving physical function
   - Resolving an infection
   - Removing a source of inflammation
   - Bringing back heart function

   Sometimes there can be multiple goals.

2. Are there other ways to achieve the desired objective? Examples include:

- Other medications with similar effects
- Medication instead of surgery

3. Does the goal coincide with what the patient wants? Examples include:
   - A cancer patient wanting only comfort care
   - An elderly patient who is DNR

Consider the Whole Patient

Take your patient's situation as a whole. Like the process of finding a diagnosis, **see the big picture and the context** of the patient's situation. In short, think of the entire patient.

Because there are many aspects to being a patient, your plan must work medically, psychologically, and socially.

Consider the Consequences of the Treatment

A good start is to ask what would happen if you did nothing and let the disease take its natural course?[Hunkink p5] This can provide a baseline from which to compare different treatment options.

Every treatment will have effects outside of its intended ones. These can be wide-ranging and can include:

- Opportunity costs (for example time, energy, and money)
- Physical injury
- Emotional costs
- Financial costs
- Lost time

Therefore, we must be mindful that our treatment plans affect more than just the patient. Depending on the situation, you may have to consider effects on the patient's family, community, or even society as a whole.

Base the Plan on Evidence

Make sure there is evidence that your plan has a good chance of working.

Thankfully, modern science provides us with lots of evidence to draw from. Use medical literature to find options for your patient's treatment. Then pick the therapy with the best evidence to support it. Since other resources cover the use of evidence-based medicine in clinical practice, I will not explore it in further detail. See the bibliography for some of these resources.

Patient Autonomy

When in doubt, involve the patient in the decision making. Discuss the options with your patient.

Patient autonomy does not mean that the patient can choose whatever testing or treatment is possible. Instead, it means that you, the clinician, use your medical knowledge and decision making skills to eliminate choices that are clearly harmful and clearly wasteful. You narrow the choices down to a set of safe options that all have a reasonable amount of benefit. Then, offer those options to the patient and let them choose, based on their individual situation and values.

When offering our patients these options, be aware of the biases and values that every medical professional brings into the situation, and how they may interact with the patient's own biases and values. The discussion of biases is too nuanced for this book, but is a topic that you will come across often as you go through your career.

Finally, ask yourself if your plan is:

1. **Logical**
2. **Safe for the patient** (medically, socially, and psychologically)

There are a range of treatment categories depending on specialty. These categories can include medications, procedures, physical therapy, cognitive-behavioral therapy, etc. One example will illustrate some important factors to consider in any treatment plan: medication.

You are selecting a new medication for a patient. At first glance, this seems pretty easy. You've seen experienced clinicians do this with ease many times. Sometimes their decision seems instantaneous. They seem to make the correct choice quickly and effortlessly. For these expert clinicians, choosing a medication is a well-practiced skill. Over time a clinician becomes an expert by using similar medications in similar situations many times. Expertise is basically having and using a well-practiced, but **implicit,** heuristic.

However, it is useful to break the process down **explicitly** for both a trainee and an expert who is prescribing a medication for the first time. Below is a list of things to consider, using the following scenario:

Example—Medical treatment: A 60-year-old female with muscular back pain. We are considering starting her on naproxen, an NSAID. The application of the questions to the specific example will be *in italics*.

How effective is the medication for the patient's condition?

- If the medication is very effective, the decision is easy. But what if the medication has a small benefit? A medium benefit?
- *Naproxen works well for muscular pain.*

What are the medication's side effects?

- Every medication has both positive and negative effects. The negative effects may outweigh the positive effects, depending on the context of the situation.
- *Naproxen's side effects include gastric irritation and renal injury.*
- *We should make sure our patient has no preexisting gastric or renal problems, or risk of such problems.*

What are the patient's medical problems?

- The new medication may worsen the patient's pre-existing medical problems.
- *If this patient has gastric ulcers or renal disease, naproxen might be a bad idea, as we mentioned above.*

What are the patient's allergies?

- If the patient has an allergy to medication of a similar class, then they may be allergic to this medication as well.
- *If the patient is allergic to an NSAID, then she should <u>not</u> use naproxen.*

- *We should check if she has had a reaction to other NSAIDs like ibuprofen or ketorolac.*

Has the patient used this medication (or a similar one) before?

- Always check with the patient to see if they taken this medication or something similar before. The patient may have a similar reaction, good or bad.
- *Other common medications in this drug family include ibuprofen and ketorolac.*
- *We should specifically ask her if she has taken these medications before. Sometimes, asking for the same information in a different way may elicit a different response.*

What medications does the patient already take?

- Medications interact with each other. Check for possible interactions.
- *Blood thinners like warfarin can interact with naproxen and increase the risk of bleeding.*
- *We should ascertain if she is on blood thinners, even though we asked previously about medical problems. Again, asking for the same information in a different way may elicit a different response.*

Who is giving the patient the medication, and how is the medication administered?

- Medications can be oral, rectal, topical, intravenous, intranasal, intramuscular, or subcutaneous.
- *Naproxen is taken by mouth. For most patients this is no problem. It may still be a good idea to see if she has a problem swallowing tablets.*

- Is the chosen administration method practical for the patient?
- *The patient or a caretaker may administer Naproxen.*

Is the medication schedule convenient for the patient?

- Once daily is easier for most people. But what if the dosing schedule is 4 or 5 times a day? This could be difficult for the patient to remember or impractical for the patient's daily schedule.
- *We should check to see if that schedule is impractical for the patient. If so, we should ask what is practical and try to find the next best alternative.*

How much does the medication cost?

- If the patient cannot afford the medication, the patient might as well not have the medication. In those cases, we should consider the next best alternative in terms of cost.
- *Naproxen is affordable for most patients. However, if we consider a costlier medication, then we should ask about her insurance or her ability to pay out of pocket.*

What alternatives are there to this medication?

- Is there an alternative that is:
    - Cheaper?
    - More effective?
    - Less likely to have side effects?
    - More convenient in terms of dosing schedule?
    - Less likely to interfere with the medications the patient already takes?

- Less likely to worsen the patient's pre-existing problems?

Lots of factors come into play for what seems like a straightforward decision at first glance. With practice and familiarity, you can quickly and easily make a decision that is equally as complex. A clinician can become an expert in using a specific medication in a certain set of circumstances.

However, an expert's expertise is domain specific.[Newell p196] **Outside of our familiar fields, all of us are novices.** Understanding the processes behind making a plan can help us navigate when we unexpectedly find ourselves in an unfamiliar circumstance.

Communicating Your Decision Making

Medical professionals transmit knowledge in two ways: **verbal** and **written** communications. I will touch on both shortly, but first I will discuss some general concepts of communication.

Because we work with others, we often have to communicate relevant information. This information is the product of our knowledge-work: our findings, our thought processes, and our conclusions. The recipients are often other knowledge-workers: clinicians, nurses, physical therapists, speech therapists, radiology technicians, social workers, etc. They need the information we give them in order to do their jobs effectively. Although obvious at first glance, clinicians easily lose sight of this fundamental concept.

4 General Tips:

1. *Beware of The Curse of Knowledge.* The Curse of Knowledge is a term that describes forgetting that your audience does not know what you already know.[Pinker ch. 3] Do not communicate with your audience as if they already know what you know. They do not know what has gone on. This is like telling an inside joke to someone who is on the outside. It is poor communication.

    If your audience does not yet know anything about the patient, then your communication should fill in the relevant gaps in the background information. **Give your audience that necessary background.**

2. *Focus on the Story You're Telling.* You should have developed a pretty good idea of what is going on

with the patient by the time you are communicating it to someone else. **Keep that diagnosis in your mind as you communicate.**

You will have accumulated a lot of data about the patient during the history, physical examination, and testing. Furthermore, you have produced *knowledge work*, or the result of your interpreted data. But not all of this data is directly relevant to the patient's story. **You are not just giving them data. You are giving them the product of your knowledge work: <u>useful information</u>.**

Tell your story in an organized and logical way. Make it easy for your audience to understand. Your audience should readily grasp what you are trying to tell them. Ideally, the conclusion should be obvious in the way that you present your story.

3. *Remember Your Audience.* Different audience members require different information. Tailor the communication to those aspects of the patient's story that the other person needs to know. Who are you communicating with:
     - The senior resident?
     - The attending?
     - A specialist consultant?
     - The nurse?
     - The respiratory therapist?
     - The social worker?
     - The patient?
     - The patient's family?
   Each one of these people will need information on different aspects of the patient's situation.

Expressing the same information in the same way to each of them is poor communication.

4. *Balance Telling Too Little and Telling Too Much.* Your audience will need some background about the patient. On the one hand, it is possible to drown them in unnecessary details. On the other hand, if you are too brief, you will not tell parts of the story that your audience needs to know for their part of the patient's care.

If you are mindful that you have to strike a balance between too little and too much information, you will get better at this quicker.

Verbal Communication

This example should solidify the concepts discussed above:

Your patient, Mr. X is a 55-year-old male with a history of hypertension, high cholesterol, and arthritis. He takes metoprolol, simvastatin, and aspirin. He is on his second day of admission for pneumonia. He is receiving IV antibiotics. At about 5 AM, he tries to get up to walk to the bathroom, slips, strikes his head, has loss of consciousness for a few moments, and thevnurses find him on the floor complaining of headache and dizziness. CT scan of his head shows left sided subarachnoid hemorrhage without midline shift. He has a normal neurological exam. You have to communicate with several people about Mr. X.

When getting ready to communicate with someone else regarding your patient, take time to **consider the information that <u>they</u> will need** in order to do their part of patient care. You are telling much of **the same information, but in a different way to each person, depending on their needs or duties**:

> *To your medical attending:* "Doctor M, Mr. X, the 55-year-old gentleman with pneumonia, had a slip and fall at 5AM this morning with a head injury. CT scan showed he had a subarachnoid hemorrhage. He only complains of headache and diffuse dizziness. On exam, he has cranial nerves normal, normal strength in all four extremities, and he's not confused. I'm going to contact neurosurgery and the ICU."

> *To the neurosurgeon:* "Doctor N, I am consulting you regarding Mr. X. He's a 55-year-old male with subarachnoid hemorrhage after a trip and fall today at about 5AM. We got a CT scan that shows a left sided subarachnoid hemorrhage without midline shift. He's taking aspirin. He's got dizziness, a diffuse headache, and had a brief loss of consciousness. On exam, he has cranial nerves 2-12 intact, 5 out of 5 strength in all 4 extremities, and recalls the event clearly. His initial admission was for pneumonia. His medical problems include hypertension, high cholesterol, and arthritis."

> *To the ICU nurse:* (on arrival to the ICU) "This is Mr. X. He's the gentleman with the subarachnoid hemorrhage after a slip and fall this morning. I know you already got report from the nurse on the medical floor. He's still oriented to person, place, and time, has cranial nerves 2-12 intact, and has 5/5 strength in all 4 extremities. His medical attending is Dr. M, and Dr. N from neurosurgery is following as a consult."

> *To the CT technician:* "I just placed the order for Mr. X's repeat CT scan. He's the patient that had a

subarachnoid hemorrhage earlier today. We need a repeat scan to see if there's been interval change. He's conversant, following commands, and stable for transport. I'll be coming to radiology with him shortly."

To Mr. X's wife: "Mrs. X, Mr. X had a slip and fall today and had a pretty bad injury to his head. He has bleeding inside of his brain, but he's stable and talking to us. We've moved him to the intensive care unit so that we can monitor his progress more closely. We also called a specialist to come and see him."

Imagine if you had communicated with each of those people using the same words. What would the quality or utility of that communication be? It does not make sense to describe one situation in the same manner to each member of the audience; they all have different needs and interact with the patient in a different way. The takeaway is this:

Tailor your communication to your audience.

Written Communication: Medical Charting

This section is not meant to be a comprehensive discussion of medical charting; however, I will introduce a few tools that will help make your medical charting better. For works about better medical charting, see the recommended resources after the bibliography.

Written communication is not just verbal communication put into writing. Think of written and verbal communication as different dialects of the same language. The same principles of communication apply. However, there are some extra concepts to keep in mind for writing.

For our examples, I will use the same case study of Mr. X, the hypothetical patient with the subarachnoid hemorrhage.

3 General Tips:

1. Omit Needless Words

   Only use necessary details in your prose. When you use too many unnecessary words, you lose your story in details that do not drive your story forward. Instead, they distract from the essentials. For instance, compare the first ICU admission note to the second:

   Needless words: Mr. X is a 55-year-old male with a history of HTN, hyperlipidemia, and arthritis. He was initially admitted for pneumonia and was on day 2 of IV antibiotics. He was progressing well. At 5 AM this morning, he had a slip and fall while walking to the bathroom in the dark. Nurses found him on the floor. He was awake and alert, but complained of a headache and dizziness. We decided to do a CT scan of his head to rule out intracranial bleed. Our CT scan showed a left sided subarachnoid hemorrhage without midline shift. We consulted neurosurgery. We transferred him to the ICU. Currently he continues to have headache, dizziness, productive cough, fever, body aches, and knee pain.

   Omitted needless words: Mr. X is a 55-year-old male with a history of HTN, hyperlipidemia, and arthritis. Originally admitted for pneumonia and receiving IV antibiotics. Slipped and fell with head injury at 5AM today. CT head showed left sided subarachnoid hemorrhage without midline shift. Neurosurgery consulted. Transferred to ICU. Currently notes headache and dizziness. Refer to review of systems for further symptoms.

2. Use the Active Voice

    Put the actor first and the acted upon second. This pattern is easier for your reader to read and understand. Ease for your reader makes for better communication.

    Avoid the passive voice, its opposite.

    Active Voice:

    I consulted Dr. N.

    Nurses found Mr. X on the floor.

    Passive Voice:

    A consult was made to Dr. N.

    Mr. X was found on the floor by nurses.

3. Pay Attention to Your Formatting

    How you lay out your words can make them easier or more difficult to understand. Because of that, you can inadvertently hide important details or explicitly highlight them through some basic formatting. **Consider what your prose will look like when you are finished writing it.** Think about how you can make it easier to read.

Pre-formatting: Mr. X is a 55-year-old male with a history of HTN, hyperlipidemia, and arthritis. Admitted for pneumonia and receiving IV antibiotics. Slipped and fell with head injury at 5AM today. CT head showed left sided subarachnoid hemorrhage without midline shift. Dr. N consulted. Transferred to ICU. Currently notes headache and dizziness. Refer to review of systems for further symptoms.

Post-formatting: Mr. X is a 55-year-old male with a history of HTN, hyperlipidemia, and arthritis. Admitted for pneumonia and receiving IV antibiotics.

Slipped and fell with head injury at 5AM today. CT head showed left sided subarachnoid hemorrhage without midline shift. Dr. N consulted. Transferred to ICU.

Currently notes headache and dizziness. Refer to review of systems for further symptoms.

Keeping all of the information in one large paragraph makes it more difficult to read. Separating the information into paragraphs that address different aspects of the case makes it easier to read.

<u>Final Notes</u>

The method I've shown you is just the basic aspects of my way. Other methods exist. If you find that those other ways work better for you, then by all means use them. Think of my way as one of many possible beginnings of your journey into becoming a clinician who makes rational clinical decisions. Try my methods and others that you will come across as you progress in your career, and then **put them together in a way that works <u>for you</u>**. The most important thing is to remember:

- You have to look for clinical decision making methods
- Put them into practice
- Try to improve yourself as a clinician

Good luck.

<u>Acknowledgements</u>

Special thanks to the following people to helped me with this book at its many stages of development:

Tamara Fish

Ilia Iliev, MD

Michael Keenaghan, MD

Adam Kramer, MD

Tanya Pohl, JD

Brian Pritchard, MD

Phillip Tan

Mollie Williams, MD

Bibliography

1. Confucius. *The Wisdom of Confucius.* Yutang L, *Ed. And trans.* Modern Library ed. New York, NY: Random House; 1994.
2. Drucker PF. *Management, Revised Edition.* ePub edition. New York, NY: HarperCollins; 2008.
3. Hunkink MG, Weinstein MC, Wittenberg E, et al. *Decision Making in Health and Medicine: Integrating Evidence and Values.* 2nd ed. Cambridge, UK: Cambridge University Press; 2014.
4. Kassirer J, Wong J, Kopelman R. *Learning Clinical Reasoning.* 2nd ed. Baltimore: MD: Lippincott Williams & Wilkins; 2010.
5. Merriam SB, Bierema L. *Adult Learning: Linking Theory and Practice.* San Francisco, CA: Wiley & Sons; 2014.
6. Newell BR, Lagnado DA, Shanks DR. *Straight Choices: The Psychology of Decision Making.* 2nd ed. East Sussex, UK: Psychology Press; 2015.
7. Pinker S. *The Sense of Style.* New York, NY: Penguin Group; 2014.
8. Sox HC, Blatt MA, Higgins MC, Marton KI. *Medical Decision Making.* Philadelphia, PA: American College o Physicians
9. Weingart S, Wyer P. *Emergency Medicine Decision Making: Critical Choices in Chaotic Environments.*

Helpful Books for Medical Charting

1. The Handbook of Medical Charting
    by Marco Tan
2. The Elements of Style
    by E.B. White and William Strunk

Printed in Great Britain
by Amazon